The Most Helpful Gout Diet Recipes

Inflammation-reducing and Gout Friendly Cookbook

BY: Valeria Ray

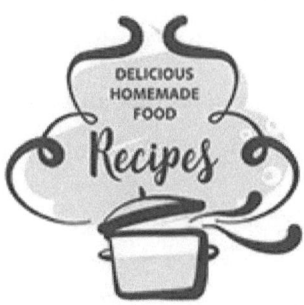

License Notes

A Special Reward for Purchasing My Book!

Thank you, cherished reader, for purchasing my book and taking the time to read it. As a special reward for your decision, I would like to offer a gift of free and discounted books directly to your inbox. All you need to do is fill in the box below with your email address and name to start getting amazing offers in the comfort of your own home. You will never miss an offer because a reminder will be sent to you. Never miss a deal and get great deals without having to leave the house! Subscribe now and start saving!

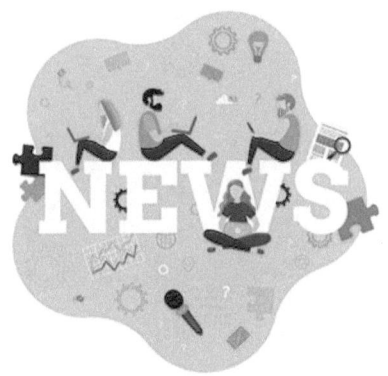
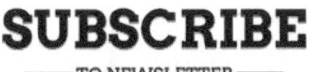

https://valeria-ray.gr8.com

Contents

Amazing Gout Diet Recipes

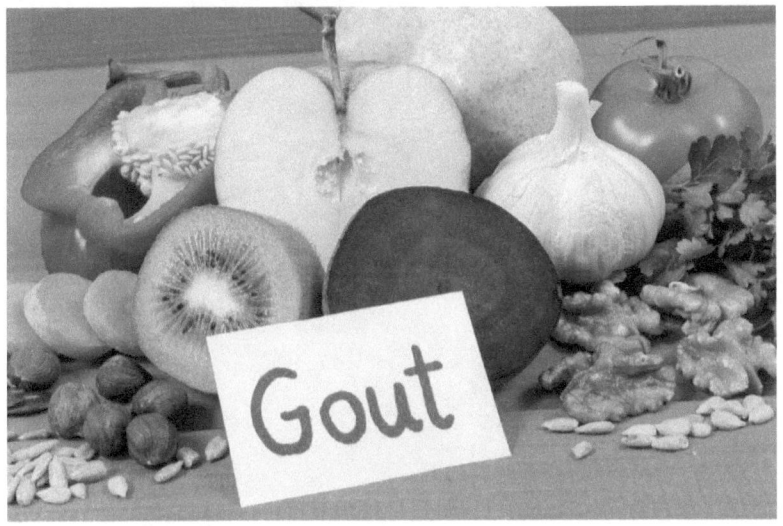

MMMMMMMMMMMMMMMMMMMMMMMMMMMMMMMMMMM

(1) Nutty Grilled Tofu

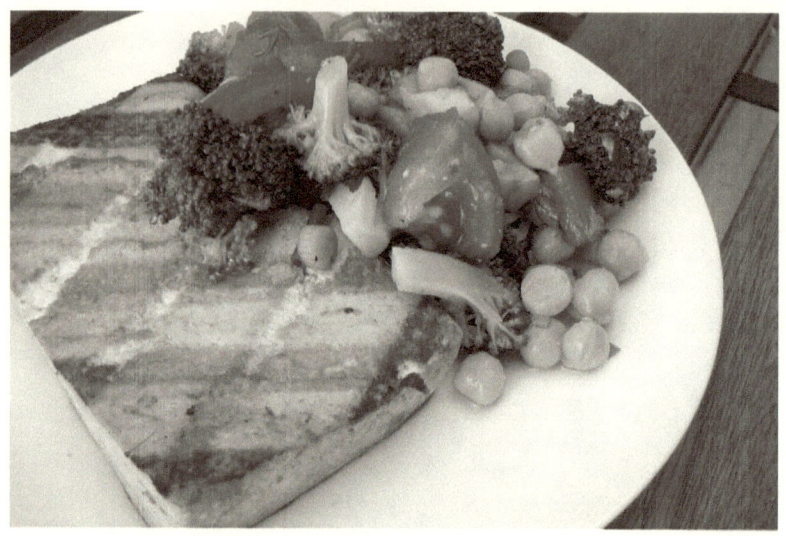

Tofu is an amazing meat substitute and this dish proves that it can be tasty, too!

Yield: 4

Total Prep Time: 1 hr. 20 mins.

List of Ingredients:

- 1 lb tofu
- 1 tablespoon brown sugar
- 2 Tablespoons soy sauce
- ¼ cup vegetable broth
- 2 Tablespoons orange juice concentrate
- Sliced scallion
- ¼ teaspoons ground ginger
- 2 Tablespoons peanut butter

MMMMMMMMMMMMMMMMMMMMMMMMMMMMMMMMMM

Methods:

1. Cut the tofu into ½ inch thick triangular shaped pieces.

2. Marinate the tofu for at least an hour in soy sauce together with brown sugar and orange juice then grill until browned.

3. Puree the peanut butter, vegetable broth, ginger and brown sugar altogether.

4. Place sliced scallions on top of the tofu then serve with a drizzle of peanut sauce. Enjoy!

(2) Chicken Cacciatore

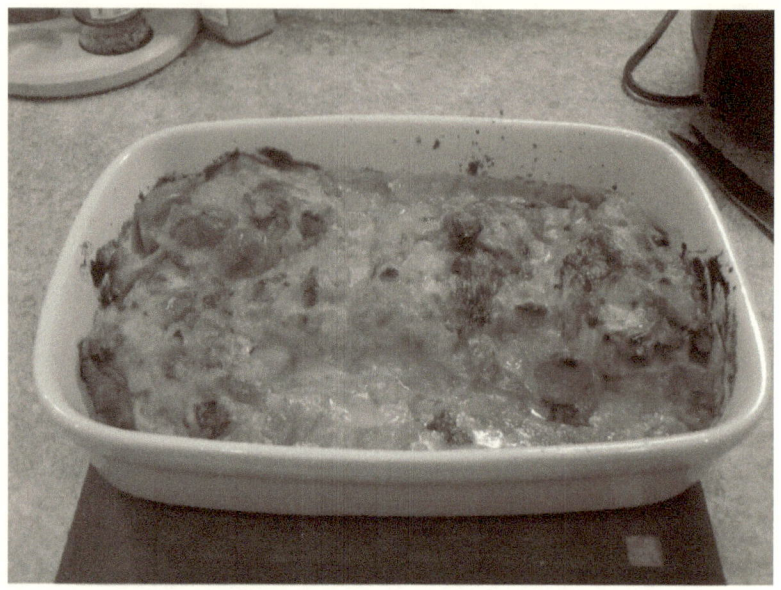

This chicken cacciatore recipe is just a burst of flavour that you cannot deny.

Yield: 6

Total Prep Time: 1 hr. 10 mins.

List of Ingredients:

- 1 tablespoon balsamic vinegar
- ½ teaspoon brown sugar
- 1 large onion, chopped
- 6 chicken thighs, skin on
- 125g button mushrooms, sliced
- 2 carrots, chopped
- 1 bay leaf
- 3 garlic, crushed
- 2 celery sticks, chopped
- 150g sliced pancetta, chopped
- 100ml white wine
- 150ml chicken stock
- 800g can diced tomatoes
- Chopped parsley
- 3 tablespoons olive oil
- 1 cup pitted Kalamata olives
- 1 tablespoon chopped fresh rosemary
- 6 chicken drumsticks, trimmed of excess fat, skin on

MMMMMMMMMMMMMMMMMMMMMMMMMMMMMMMM

Methods:

1. In a large casserole dish, heat the oil over medium-high heat. Place the pieces of chicken in the casserole dish and cook until it is fully browned.

2. Once the chicken is browned. Transfer the chicken to a plate. Add pancetta, carrot, celery and onion to the pan and cook for 5 minutes over low heat.

3. Add the mushrooms and garlic and cook for a minute.

4. Return the seared chicken pieces back in the casserole dish. Add the white wine in the pan and let it simmer for about 2 minutes.

5. Add the stock, tomatoes, vinegar, sugar and herbs. Bring the contents in the pan to a boil, reduce the heat to low. Cover the pan and let cook for twenty minutes, stir often.

6. Add the kalamata and let it cook for another 10 minutes.

7. Take the chicken out, over high heat for 6 minutes reduces the sauce. Use the parsley to garnished and serve.

(3) Tomato and Macaroni Salad

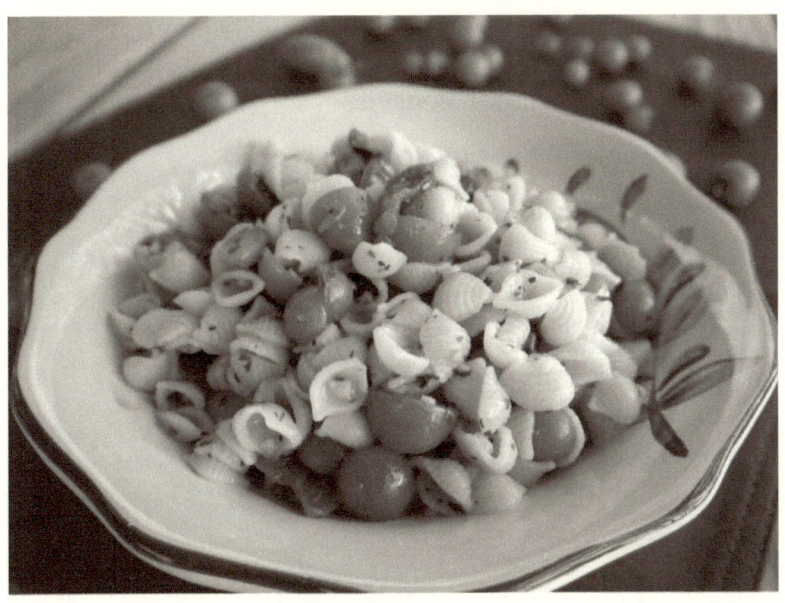

You can never go wrong with this classic.

Yield: 4

Total Prep Time: 6 mins.

List of Ingredients:

- 4 medium tomatoes, diced
- ½ cup fresh basil, chopped finely
- 3 cups macaroni, cooked
- 4 Tablespoons olive oil
- 2 cloves garlic, crushed
- ¾ teaspoons salt
- 2 Tablespoons vinegar
- ½ teaspoons pepper

MMMMMMMMMMMMMMMMMMMMMMMMMMMMMMMMM

Methods:

1. Combine macaroni, tomatoes and basil in a bowl then set aside.

2. Combine the rest of the ingredients in another bowl then pour over the macaroni and tomato mixture.

3. Toss until well-combined then serve in bowls. Enjoy!

(4) Gout Friendly Breakfast Cereal Bowl

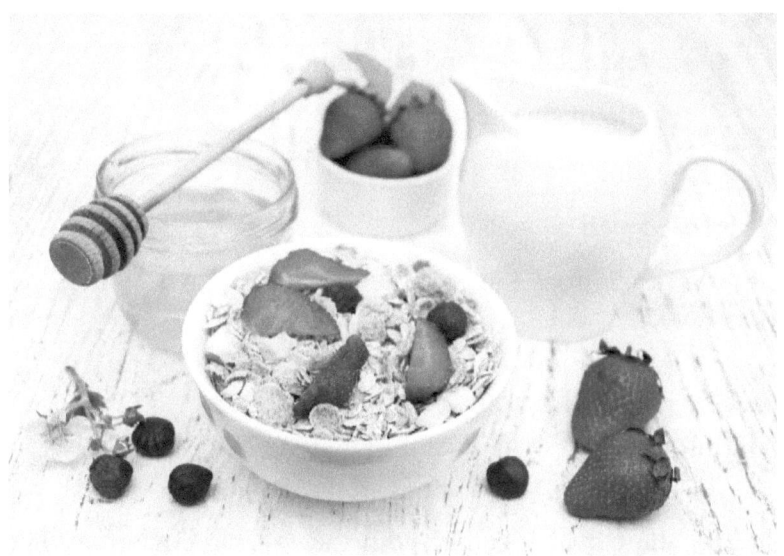

This recipe helps you create a delicious breakfast bowl that is great in the fight against inflammation and a brilliant start to your day.

Yield: 1

Total Prep Time: 10 mins.

List of Ingredients:

- ¾ cup gluten-free cereal
- 1 tablespoon nut butter, unsweetened
- 2 Tablespoons raisins
- ¼ teaspoons ground cinnamon
- ½ cup unsweetened milk
- A pinch of salt
- ½ small banana
- 3 to 5 drops Stevia

MMMMMMMMMMMMMMMMMMMMMMMMMMMMMMMMM

Methods:

1. Mix the cereal together with the raisins, cinnamon, nut butter and salt in a bowl.

2. Place banana on top.

3. Add Stevia, if desired so milk could be sweetened and pour it all over the cereal.

4. Serve and enjoy!

(5) Meaty Cupcake with Mashed Potato Frost

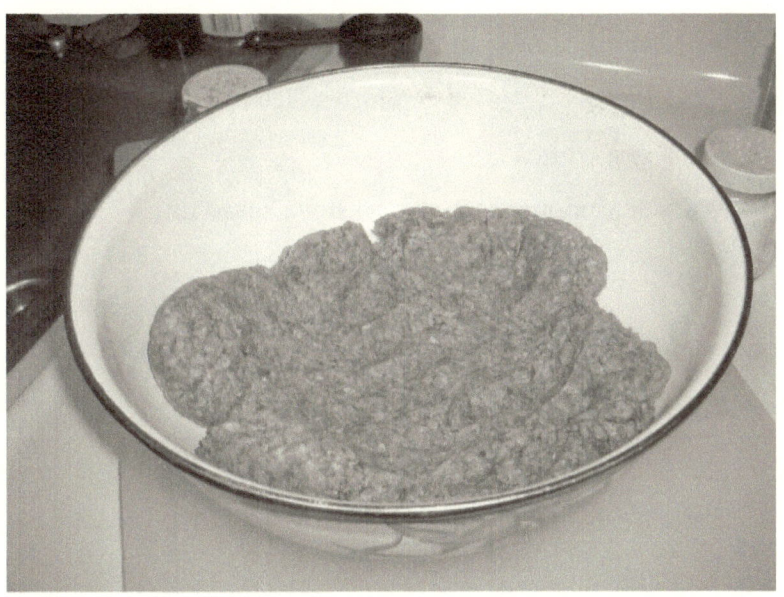

Now you'll be able to eat a dessert that's unlike any other! Aside from being safe for people with gout, this dessert is also recommended for those suffering from Crohn's disease and diabetes, as well.

Yield: 6

Total Prep Time: 45 mins.

List of Ingredients:

For the cupcakes:

- 2 lbs extra lean ground beef
- 1 cup Japanese breadcrumbs
- 1 teaspoon Worcestershire sauce
- 2 egg whites
- ¾ teaspoons less-sodium steak seasoning
- ½ medium onion, chopped finely

For the frosting:

- 3 cups potatoes, mashed
- 12 grape tomatoes
- ¼ cup reduced sodium ketchup
- 2 Tablespoons flat leaf parsley, chopped

MMMMMMMMMMMMMMMMMMMMMMMMMMMMMMMMMM

Methods:

1. Pre-heat the oven to 375 degrees.

2. Combine egg whites, seasoning, chopped onion, breadcrumbs, ground beef and Worcestershire sauce in a bowl then scoop the meat into cooking spray coated muffin tins.

3. Bake for at least 20 minutes.

4. While baking the meatloaf, prepare the frosting by placing the mashed potatoes in a re-sealable bag. Snip off a corner of the bag so piping could come out then place a meatloaf on a plate and pipe the mashed potato frost on top.

5. Sprinkle the cupcakes with parsley and serve with a drizzle of ketchup and a grape tomato on top. Enjoy!

(6) British Rumbledethumps

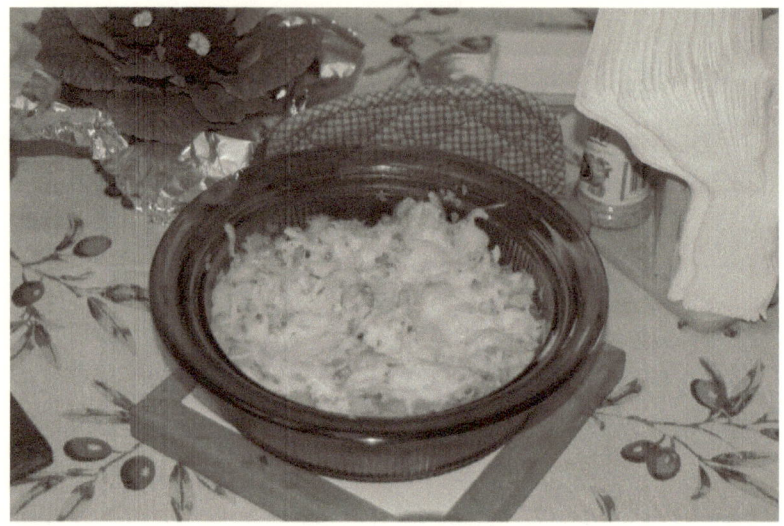

This is a healthy and delicious British vegetarian dish that is easy to whip up and can serve as a delicious alternative to a casserole or lasagne.

Yield: 6

Total Prep Time: 45 mins.

List of Ingredients:

- 1 lb green cabbage
- 1 lb potato, sliced
- 3 oz nut butter
- 2 leeks, chopped finely
- 2 oz cheddar cheese
- Light cream (1 cup)
- Salt (to taste)
- Black pepper (to taste)
- Fresh chives, chopped

MMMMMMMMMMMMMMMMMMMMMMMMMMMMMMMMM

Methods:

1. Boil the potato in salted water then drain and mash afterwards.

2. Next, slice the cabbage then steam it in salted water and make sure not to overcook.

3. Melt butter then cook with leeks.

4. Once the leeks are soft and the butter is melted, add the cabbage and the potatoes together with cream. Season to taste and beat until well-blended.

5. Put the mixture in an oven-safe dish then add cheddar cheese on top and broil until browned.

6. Serve garnished with fresh chives and enjoy!

(7) Dreamy Coco Pie

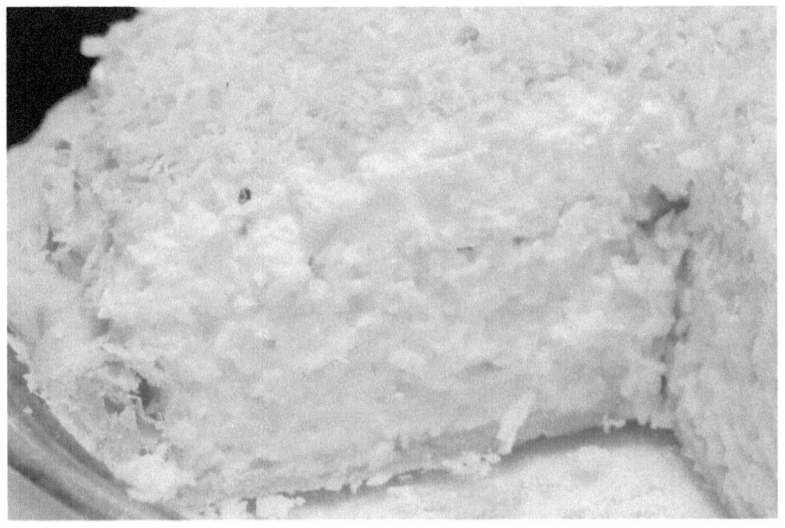

A cake that's sure to keep you coming back for more!

Yield: 10

Total Prep Time: 4 hrs. 8 mins.

List of Ingredients:

- 2 ¾ cups skim milk
- 2 envelopes Kraft topping mix
- 1 teaspoon coconut extract
- 1 teaspoon vanilla extract
- 1 graham cracker crust
- 1 cup coconut, toasted
- 2 boxes fat-free vanilla pudding mix

MMMMMMMMMMMMMMMMMMMMMMMMMMMMMMMMMM

Methods:

1. Beat the Kraft topping mix together with vanilla and a cup of milk until very stiff or for around 6 minutes using an electric mixer.

2. Add the remaining milk and Kraft topping mix together with coconut extract and beat for around 2 minutes and then fold coconut into the pie shell.

3. Chill for around 4 hours then serve topped with extra coconut curls. Enjoy!

(8) Healthy Easy French Toast

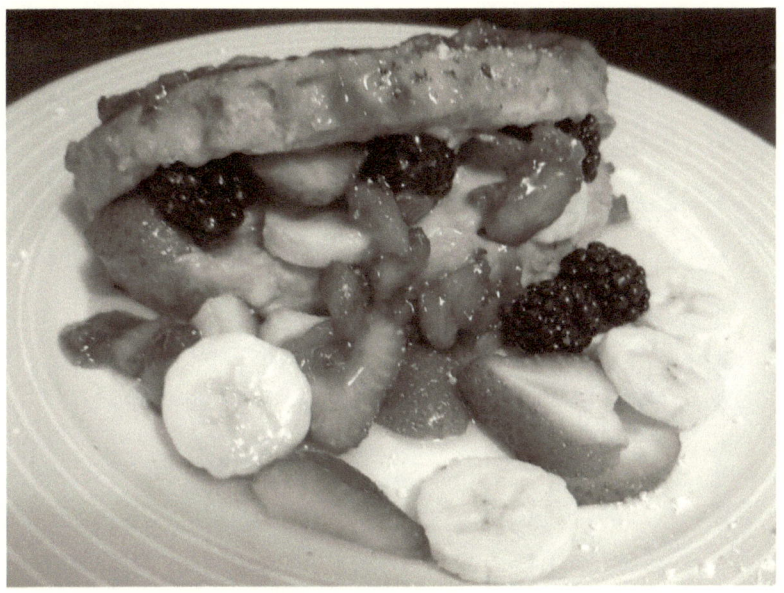

This is a healthy take on this breakfast classic.

Yield: 2

Total Prep Time: 18 mins.

List of Ingredients:

- ¾ cup low fat milk
- 8 slices whole wheat bread
- 1 large egg
- ½ teaspoons salt
- 2 teaspoons butter
- ¼ teaspoons vanilla extract
- 2 large egg whites

MMMMMMMMMMMMMMMMMMMMMMMMMMMMMMM

Methods:

1. Pre-heat the oven at 200 degrees.

2. Whisk milk, egg, salt and egg whites in a pie plate together with vanilla then whisk until well-combined. Then, melt a teaspoon of butter in a pan over medium heat.

3. Dip bread in the mixture a piece at a time then cook each side for 3 to 4 minutes or until lightly browned.

4. Transfer the bread onto a cookie sheet then place in the oven to keep warm. Repeat with the remaining bread slices and egg and milk mixture.

5. Serve warm and enjoy! You may also serve this topped with your choice of fruit, if desired. Best choices include strawberries or mangoes.

(9) Sweet Raspberry Tarts

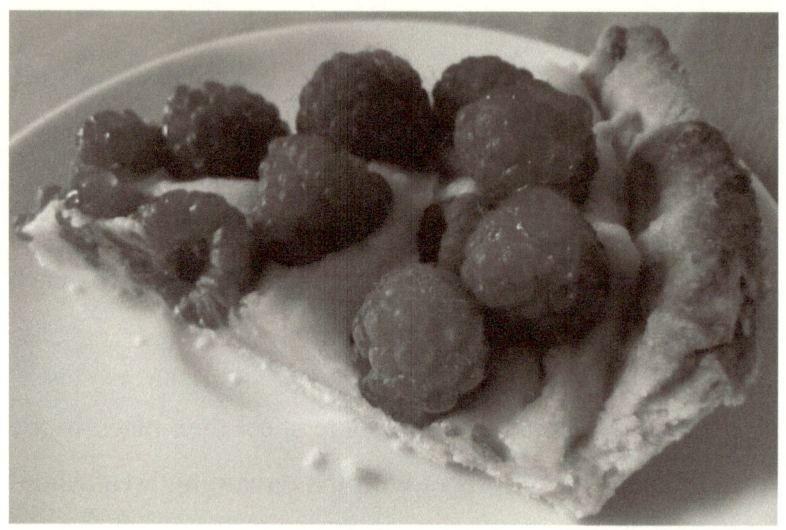

For me, this sweet tartness of raspberries is pretty irresistible.

Yield: 10

Total Prep Time: 30 mins.

List of Ingredients:

- 1 pack block-style cream cheese
- 1 pack sugar cookie dough, refrigerated
- Fresh raspberries
- ½ teaspoons vanilla extract
- Zest of 1 orange
- ¼ cup sugar

MMMMMMMMMMMMMMMMMMMMMMMMMMMMMMMMM

Methods:

1. Pre-heat the oven to 350 degrees then coat a muffin tin with cooking spray.

2. Divide the cookie dough into 32 pieces then coat your hands in flour and make balls out of the dough.

3. Press the balls into the muffin tin one by one then form tart-shaped pieces out of them.

4. Bake until golden or for around 10 to 12 minutes then cool in a pan for 10 more minutes.

5. Remove the tarts from cooking and let them cool on a wire rack.

6. Combine cream cheese, orange zest, sugar and vanilla in a bowl using an electric mixer.

7. Spoon the mixture into each of the tarts then top each tart with fresh raspberries.

8. Chill before serving and enjoy!

(10) Ginger, Sweet Potato and Carrot Soup

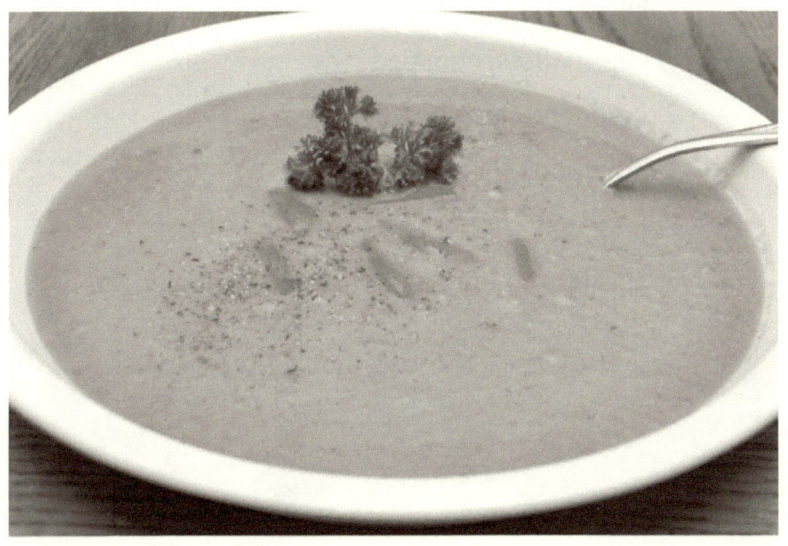

The pureed carrots make this soup creamy so there's no need to use milk or cream!

Yield: 4

Total Prep Time: 40 mins.

List of Ingredients:

- 1 ½ cups carrots, sliced and peeled
- 2 teaspoons canola oil
- 3 cups sweet potato, peeled and cubed
- ½ cup shallots, chopped
- 2 teaspoons curry powder
- 1 tablespoon ginger, grated
- ½ teaspoons salt
- 3 cups less sodium and fat-free chicken broth

MMMMMMMMMMMMMMMMMMMMMMMMMMMMMMMMM

Methods:

1. In a large saucepan, heat oil over medium heat then add shallots and sauté until tender or for at least 3 minutes.

2. Add carrots, potato, ginger and curry and cook for 2 minutes.

3. Add the broth and boil the mixture.

4. After boiling, reduce the heat and cover then simmer for at least 25 minutes then add salt and stir.

5. Place the soup in a food processor then pulse until mixture is smooth.

6. Serve topped with extra carrot shreds if desired and enjoy!

(11) Perfect Vanilla Pudding

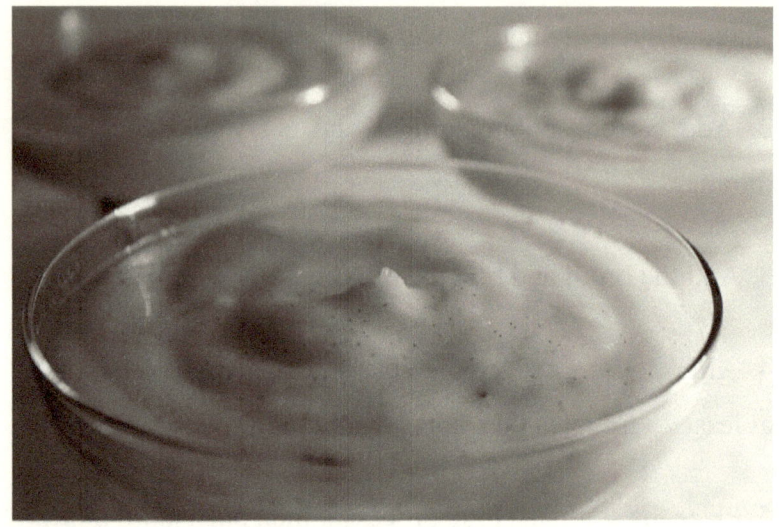

This recipe is the perfect thing for an impressive make-ahead dessert for a party.

Yield: 2

Total Prep Time: 25 mins.

List of Ingredients:

- 1 vanilla bean, split lengthwise
- 2 ½ cups reduced fat milk
- 3 Tablespoons cornstarch
- ¾ cup sugar
- 2 large egg yolks
- ¼ cup half and half
- 4 teaspoons butter
- 1/8 teaspoons salt

MMMMMMMMMMMMMMMMMMMMMMMMMMMMMMMMM

Methods:

1. Put milk in a saucepan then scrape the seeds of the vanilla bean and add both the bean and the seeds to the milk. Boil the mixture.

2. Combine cornstarch, sugar and salt in a bowl then stir well before mixing egg yolks with the half and half.

3. Add egg yolk into the sugar mixture then cook for at least a minute and stir with a whisk.

4. Remove mixture from heat then add butter and stir until butter is melted. Remove the bean and discard.

5. Spoon some of the pudding into a bowl then put the bowl in an ice-filled bowl until it cools or for around 15 minutes.

6. Make sure to stir occasionally. Cover with plastic wrap before serving and chill. Enjoy!

(12) The Best Pumpkin Pancakes

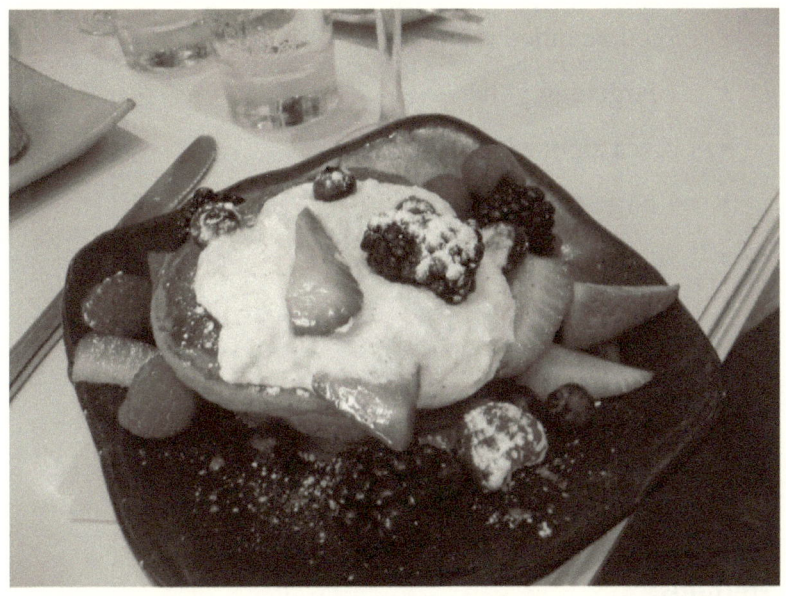

Pumpkins are actually tasty when made into pancakes and are great in regulating your digestive processes, too!

Yield: 4

Total Prep Time: 16 mins.

List of Ingredients:

- ½ cup low fat vanilla yogurt
- ½ cup canned pumpkin
- 1 large egg yolk
- ¼ teaspoons baking soda
- 4 large egg whites
- ¼ cup cake flour
- Maple syrup
- Cooking spray
- ¼ teaspoons salt

MMMMMMMMMMMMMMMMMMMMMMMMMMMMMMMM

Methods:

1. Whisk the baking soda, yogurt, pumpkin, egg yolk and flour together then whisk salt and egg whites together in another bowl, too. Fold this into the pumpkin mixture.

2. Next, coat a non-stick skillet with cooking spray and heat it over medium heat.

3. Spoon around 1/3 cup batter to make a pancake then cook for around 3 minutes each side or until lightly browned.

4. Serve with maple syrup on top, if desired.

(13) Berry Peachy Delight

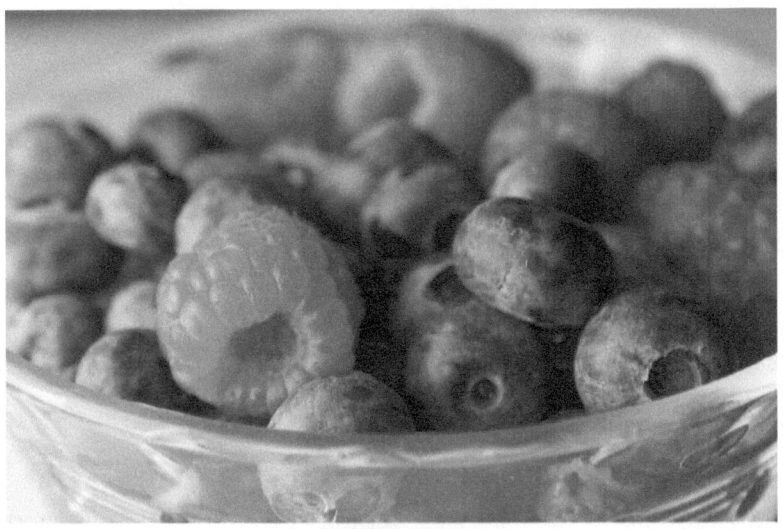

This mix of peaches and berries is truly delightful and refreshing!

Yield: 2

Total Prep Time: 5 mins.

List of Ingredients:

- 2 peaches, pitted and sliced
- ½ cup fresh strawberries
- ½ cup fresh raspberries
- 1 tablespoon fresh lemon juice
- 2 Tablespoons honey
- 2 cups vanilla low-fat ice cream

MMMMMMMMMMMMMMMMMMMMMMMMMMMMMMMMMM

Methods:

1. Combine honey, berries, lemon juice in a blender and puree until smooth. Strain through a sieve then set aside after discarding the seeds.

2. Place the peach slices into dessert bowls then add a cup of ice cream on each.

3. Serve peaches and ice cream drizzled with the berry sauce that you have made. Enjoy!

(14) Chicken Sesame

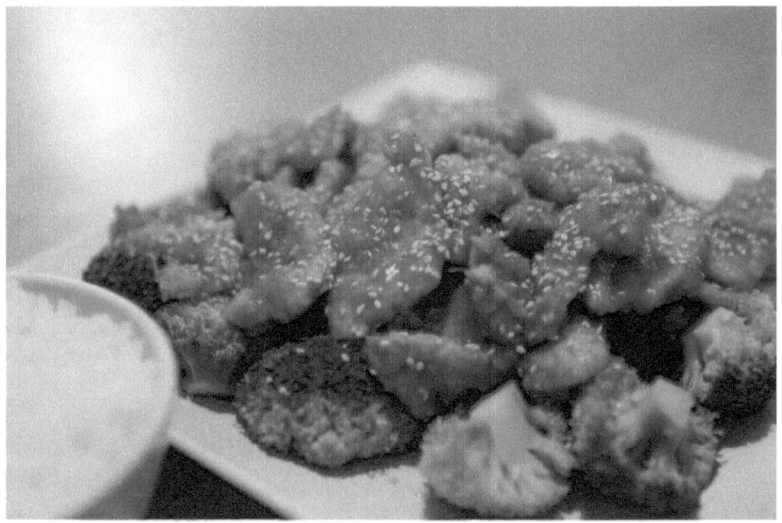

No, don't expect the cave to open up any time but expect a really tasty and nutritious Chinese-inspired dish that you'll surely love!

Yield: 6

Total Prep Time: 26 mins.

List of Ingredients:

- ½ cup honey
- 6 skinless and boneless chicken breast halves
- ½ cup soy sauce
- 1 tablespoon toasted sesame seeds
- ½ to 1 teaspoon red pepper flakes
- ½ to 1 teaspoon ground ginger
- 2 Tablespoons cornstarch
- 1 cup water

MMMMMMMMMMMMMMMMMMMMMMMMMMMMMMMM

Methods:

1. Cut the chicken breast into 1-inch thick strips then heat a skillet over medium heat.

2. Cook the chicken until it is no longer pink or for around 6 minutes then mix soy sauce, honey, cornstarch, water, red pepper flakes and ginger altogether in a bowl.

3. Whisk until there are no more lumps.

4. Pour this mixture over the chicken then cook until sauce is slightly thickened. Add more water if you feel like the sauce is too thick.

5. Sprinkle sesame seeds on top then simmer for at least 10 minutes, covered.

6. Serve with extra sesame seeds, if desired and enjoy!

(15) Oh, so Cool Yogurt Drink

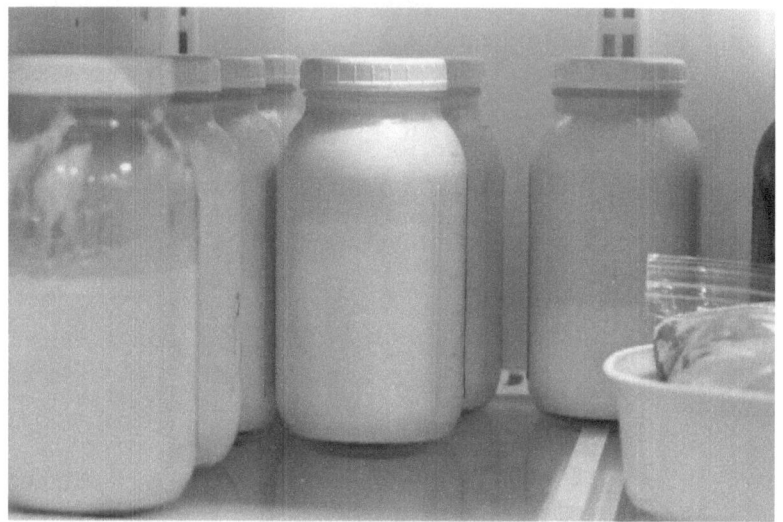

Yogurt will no longer be boring with this drink. The mint leaves make it all the cooler so it's the perfect dessert for a hot summer day!

Serving time: 2

Total Prep Time: 6 mins.

List of Ingredients:

- 2 cups water
- 5 cups low-fat yogurt
- Mint leaves, chopped finely
- Crushed ice
- 1 teaspoon salt

MMMMMMMMMMMMMMMMMMMMMMMMMMMMMMMMMM

Methods:

1. Put all of the ingredients in a blender with the exception of crushed ice and mint leaves then blend for a minute.

2. Serve the drink with crushed ice and mint leaves on top. Enjoy!

(16) Cheesy Eggplant Sandwich

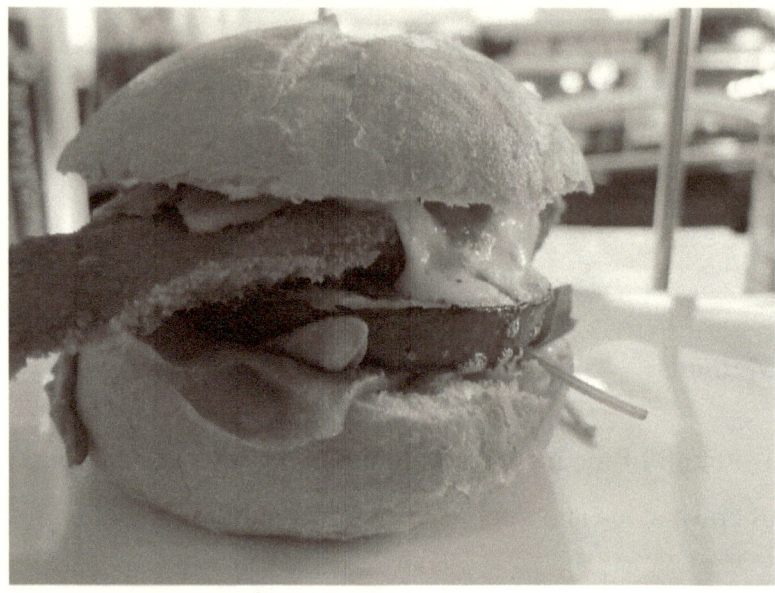

The eggplant subdues the dairy content of the goat cheese so this is good for you.

List of Ingredients:

- 2 small eggplant, cut into ¼ inch thin slices
- 1 teaspoon olive oil
- ¼ teaspoons freshly ground black pepper
- ¼ teaspoons salt
- 2 slices tomato, cut into ¼ inch pieces
- 2 rustic sandwich rolls
- ¼ cup goat cheese, softened
- Cooking spray
- ½ cup arugula

MMMMMMMMMMMMMMMMMMMMMMMMMMMMMM

Methods:

1. Pre-heat the oven to 275 degrees then brush the eggplant with oil.

2. Next, heat a non-stick skillet over medium heat then add eggplant and cook each side for 5 minutes or until lightly browned. Season with salt and pepper.

3. Spread around a tablespoon of goat cheese on one side of the sandwich rolls then place the rolls on a baking sheet with the sides with cheese on top. Bake until thoroughly heated or for 8 to 10 minutes.

4. Remove the sandwich from the oven then top each with eggplant, a slice of tomato and some arugula.

5. Serve immediately and enjoy!

(17) Yogurt Cucumber

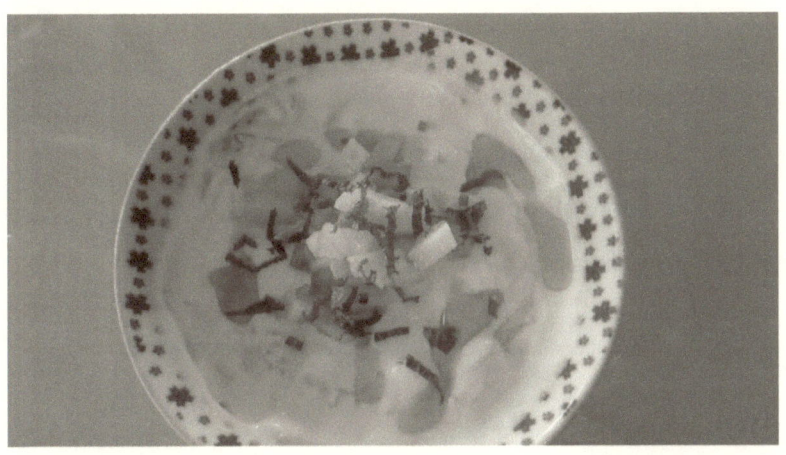

This snack will keep you feeling good and healthy!

Yield: 4

Total Prep Time: 1 hr.

List of Ingredients:

- 1 medium cucumber, peeled, quartered and sliced thinly
- 2 cups low fat yogurt
- 2 cloves garlic, crushed
- 2 Tablespoons fresh mint, chopped finely
- ½ teaspoons salt

MMMMMMMMMMMMMMMMMMMMMMMMMMMMMMMMM

Methods:

1. Put all of the ingredients in a bowl and mix until well-combined. Chill for around 30 minutes to an hour before serving and enjoy!

(18) Veggie Lasagna

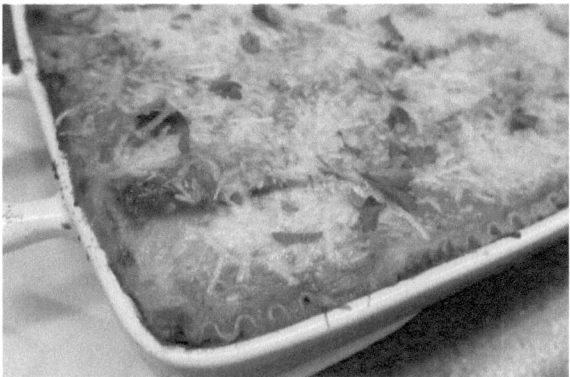

We love this recipe as much as our healthy spinach lasagna. This veggie lasagna doesn't require too much time, either.

List of Ingredients:

- ½ cup carrot, grated
- 1 ½ quarts spaghetti sauce
- ½ teaspoons oregano
- 16 oz ricotta cheese
- 6 lasagna noodles, cooked
- 2 eggs
- 1 pack frozen chopped spinach, thawed then drained well
- 3 cups part skim mozzarella cheese, shredded
- 1 cup fresh mushrooms, sliced
- ½ cup Parmesan cheese, grated
- 1 ½ cups zucchini, sliced thinly

MMMMMMMMMMMMMMMMMMMMMMMMMMMMMMM

Methods:

1. Mix the spaghetti sauce together with oregano and carrots in a bowl then mix spinach, ricotta and eggs in another bowl.

2. Spread at least ½ cup of spaghetti sauce in the bottom of a baking dish then layer 3 lasagna noodles, the remaining sauce, half of the ricotta mixture, half of the Mozzarella and half of the Parmesan and repeat process with the remaining layers.

3. Bake for around 45 minutes at 350 degrees.

4. Serve immediately and enjoy!

(19) Awesome Edamame Dumplings

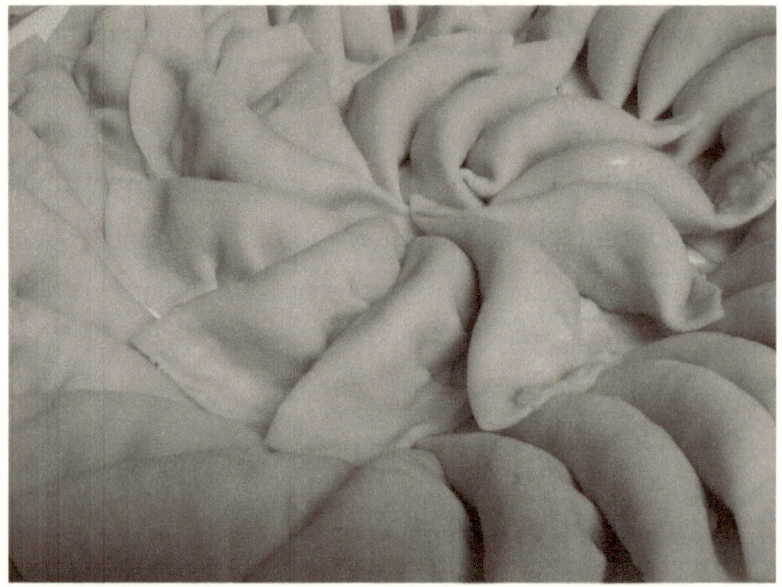

Aside from your usual meat or seafood fillings, you can actually make use of Edamame as the filling of your dumplings as they are very lean and healthy and would help you digest food easily.

Yield: 6

Total Prep Time: 17 mins.

List of Ingredients:

- 2 Tablespoons soy sauce
- 2 Tablespoons green onions, chopped
- 1 cup frozen edamame, shelled
- 1 teaspoon honey
- 1 teaspoon ground cumin
- 1 teaspoon dark sesame oil
- 1 teaspoon fresh lemon juice
- 3 garlic cloves, minced
- ½ teaspoons hot pepper flakes
- ¼ teaspoons salt
- Cooking spray
- 2 teaspoons cornstarch
- 20 wonton wrappers
- ½ cup water, divided

MMMMMMMMMMMMMMMMMMMMMMMMMMMMMMMM

Methods:

1. Combine green onions, honey and soy sauce in a small bowl to create the sauce. Stir with a whisk.

2. Cook edamame according to package directions and drain. Rinse with cold water and drain well once more. Mix edamame with juice, cumin, sesame oil, salt, garlic and red pepper flakes in a food processor. Pulse until smooth.

3. Spoon a teaspoon of the mixture into one wonton wrapper at a time then moisten the edges with water to fold. Form triangles and seal then place the dumplings on a baking sheet.

4. Heat a skillet over medium heat then coat pan with cooking spray. Arrange the dumplings in a pan then cook each side for about a minute or until lightly browned. Add water then cover and cook for 30 seconds before taking off the cover. Cook until liquid evaporates or for a minute more.

5. Repeat the process with the rest of the dumplings then serve immediately with sauce on the side or on top.

6. Enjoy!

(20) Easy Sushi

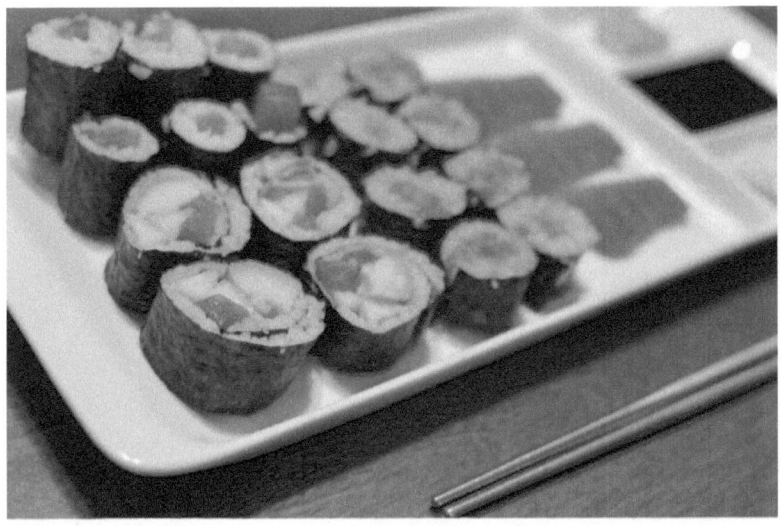

Here's light and filling Japanese dish that you'll certainly enjoy!

Yield: 4

Total Prep Time: 30 mins.

List of Ingredients:

- 1 cup freshly cooked short grain rice
- 2 Tablespoons sesame seeds, toasted
- 3 Tablespoons rice vinegar, seasoned

For the filling:

- ½ cup smoked salmon, chopped into small pieces
- 1 large ripe mango
- ¼ lb fresh small shrimp
- 1 can tuna in water
- 1 large avocado
- 1 small fresh cucumber
- Wasabi paste
- 4 oz cream cheese

MMMMMMMMMMMMMMMMMMMMMMMMMMMMMMMM

Methods:

1. Spread rice in a shallow dish and sprinkle with sesame seeds and rice vinegar. Toss gently until well-combined but make sure not to stir to avoid the rice from clumping.

2. Place at least a teaspoon of rice into your palm and create a ball out of it. Make sure to create some indents in the center with your finger.

3. Mix the ingredients for the filling in a small bowl then dip your fingers in the water and pack the rice firmly.

4. Repeat the process with the rest of the rice and the filling.

5. Sprinkle sesame seeds over the sushi balls then cover with plastic wrap and serve at room temperature.

(21) Rosemary Potatoes

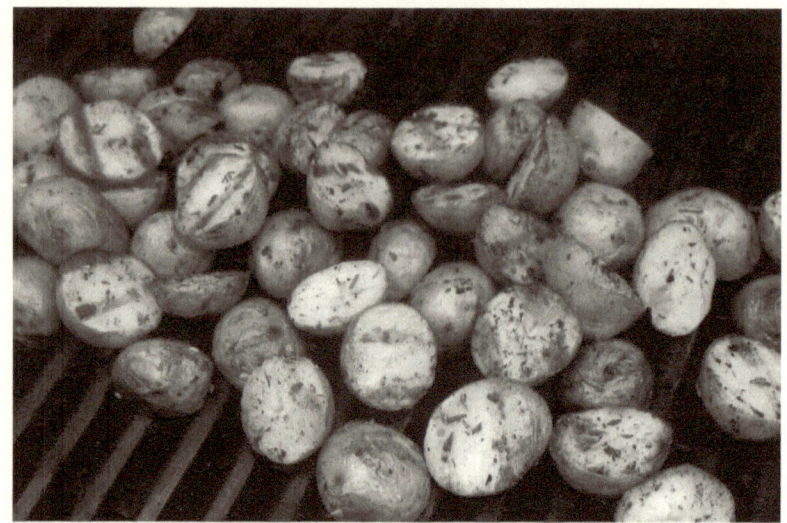

This recipe consists of potatoes roasted with rosemary! Yum!

Yield: 6

Total Prep Time: 32 mins.

List of Ingredients:

- 1 pack red potato wedges
- 3 garlic cloves, crushed
- 2 Tablespoons fresh rosemary, chopped
- ¼ teaspoons salt
- 1 tablespoon olive oil
- ¼ teaspoons pepper
- ½ teaspoons onion powder

MMMMMMMMMMMMMMMMMMMMMMMMMMMMMMMM

Methods:

1. Pre-heat the oven to 500 degrees.

2. Combine potatoes with the rest of the ingredients in a large bowl then toss thoroughly until potatoes are well-coated. Line a baking sheet with foil.

3. Arrange the potato wedges on the baking sheet.

4. Bake until golden and tender or for around 22 minutes. Serve hot and enjoy!

(22) Seedy Broccoli

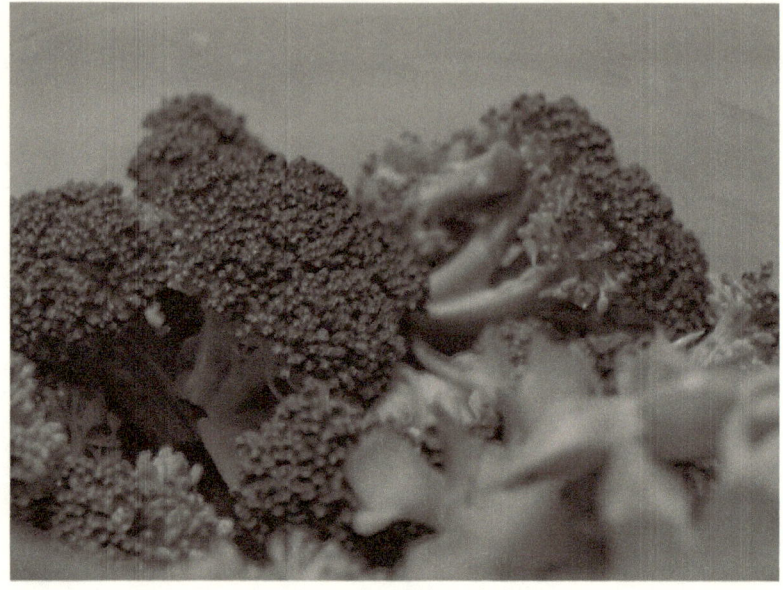

This recipe was quick and easy but more importantly, it was delicious.

Yield: 4

Total Prep Time: 16 mins.

List of Ingredients:

- 4 cups broccoli florets
- 2 teaspoons sesame seeds
- 2 Tablespoons low sodium soy sauce
- 3 Tablespoons sweet red peppers, chopped finely
- 1 tablespoon water
- ¼ teaspoons dry mustard
- ¼ teaspoons ground ginger
- 2 teaspoons sugar

MMMMMMMMMMMMMMMMMMMMMMMMMMMMMMMM

Methods:

1. Place broccoli together with the red peppers in a steamer and steam for around 5 minutes, covered. After steaming, place the vegetables in a bowl.

2. Then, heat oil in a skillet over medium heat while the vegetables are cooking. Add the sesame seeds and cook until vegetables are toasted or for around a minute. Set aside.

3. Combine water, soy sauce, sugar, mustard and ginger in a bowl and stir well.

4. Put in the microwave until bubbly or for around 45 seconds then pour the sauce over the vegetables. Toss gently and sprinkle sesame seeds on top.

(23) Potato and Garlic Mix

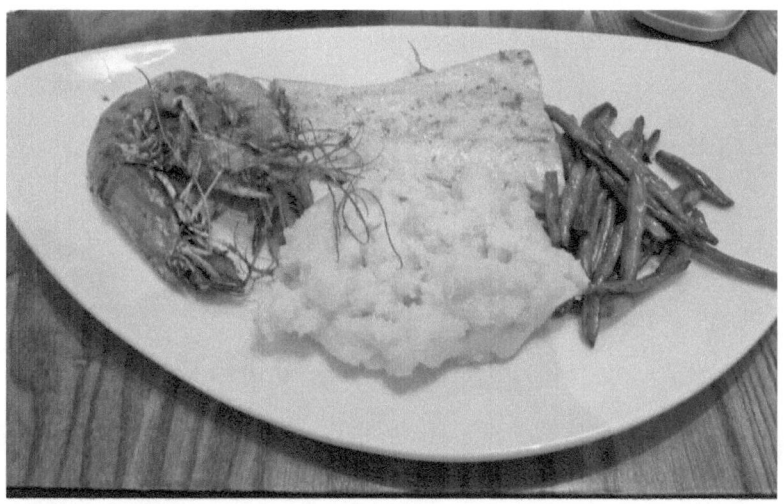

I love mashed potatoes and so does my family. It is one of our favorite sides.

Yield: 4

Total Prep Time: 10 mins.

List of Ingredients:

- 2 cups potatoes, mashed
- 6 Tablespoons olive oil
- 8 cloves garlic, crushed
- ¾ teaspoons pepper
- 1 teaspoon salt
- ½ cup plain low-fat yogurt
- 4 medium radishes, sliced
- 8 black olives, pitted and sliced in half

MMMMMMMMMMMMMMMMMMMMMMMMMMMMMMMM

Methods:

1. Combine potatoes, olive oil, garlic, salt, yogurt and pepper in a platter then serve with radishes and olives on the side. Make sure to chill before serving.

(24) Zucchini Spaghetti

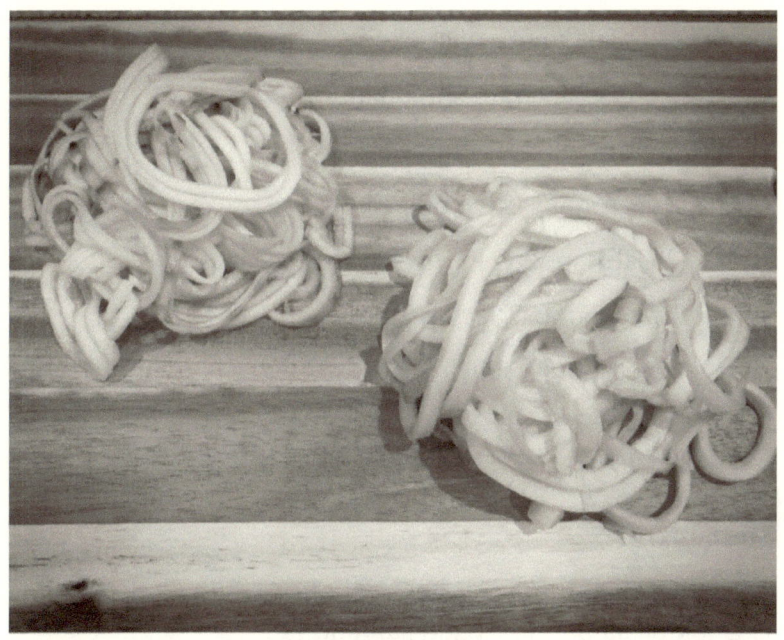

This zucchini spaghetti is a fast and simple recipe that anyone can make.

Yield: 6

Total Prep Time: 14 mins.

List of Ingredients:

- 1 can chipotle chilies
- ¾ lb spaghetti, uncooked
- 4 cups zucchini, shredded
- 2 garlic cloves, minced
- 2 teaspoons olive oil
- 2 Tablespoons Parmesan cheese, shaved
- ¼ teaspoons black pepper
- ¾ teaspoons salt

MMMMMMMMMMMMMMMMMMMMMMMMMMMMMMMMM

Methods:

1. Cook pasta but don't add salt and fat.

2. Mince the chili then heat oil in a skillet over medium heat. Add the sauce together with garlic and chili then add zucchini and cook for around 4 minutes. Make sure to stir constantly.

3. Toss zucchini and pasta together then season with cheese, salt and pepper.

4. Serve and enjoy!

(25) Plum Tomato Crostini

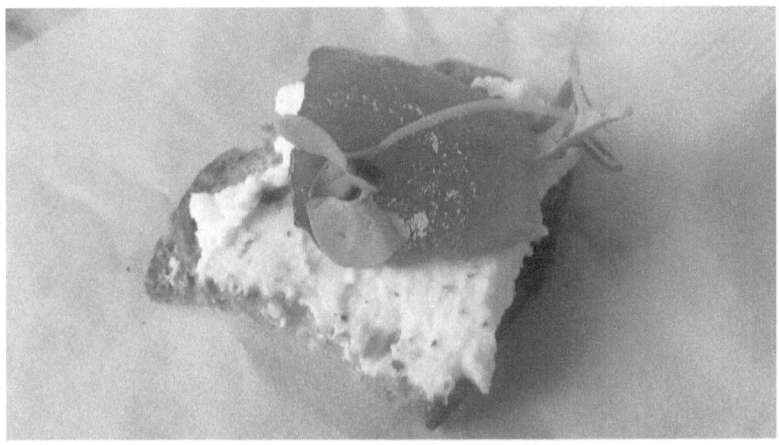

By using plum tomatoes, you can be sure that you are able to create an appetizing and flavorful snack!

Yield: 4

Total Prep Time: 18 mins.

List of Ingredients:

- 1 tablespoon fresh basil, chopped
- ½ cup plum tomato, chopped
- ½ teaspoons balsamic vinegar
- 1 teaspoon capers
- 1 tablespoon pitted green olives, chopped
- 1/8 teaspoons sea salt
- ½ teaspoons olive oil
- Cooking spray
- A dash of freshly ground black pepper
- 1 garlic clove, halved
- 4 slices French Bread Baguette

MMMMMMMMMMMMMMMMMMMMMMMMMMMMMM

Methods:

1. Pre-heat the oven to 375 degrees.

2. Combine plum tomatoes, balsamic vinegar, basil, olive oil, sea salt, capers, garlic and freshly ground black pepper in a bowl.

3. Then, coat bread slices with cooking spray and arrange them on a baking sheet. Bake until toasted or for around 4 minutes each side.

4. Serve topped with garlic and tomato mixture and enjoy!

(26) Healthy Waldorf Salad

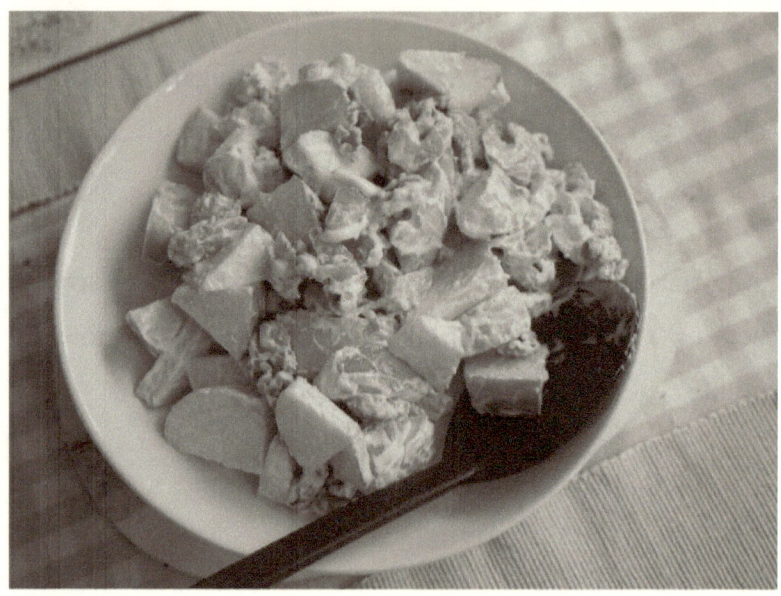

Here's a healthy take on one of the world's most popular types of salad!

Yield: 2

Total Prep Time: 2 hrs.

List of Ingredients:

- 1 tablespoon lemon juice
- 2 Tablespoons low-fat mayonnaise
- 1 cup seedless red grapes, halved
- 2 small apples, cubed
- ¼ cup celery, sliced thinly
- ¼ cup walnuts, chopped coarsely
- 1/3 cup dried cranberries
- 8 Boston lettuce leaves

MMMMMMMMMMMMMMMMMMMMMMMMMMMMMMMMM

Methods:

1. Combine lemon juice and mayonnaise in a bowl then add cranberries, grapes and apples and mix thoroughly.

2. Add celery and walnuts and mix them altogether. Serve the salad on a bed of lettuce leaves.

3. You may also refrigerate this for around 2 hours before serving, if desired. Enjoy!

(27) The Best Barbecue Wrap

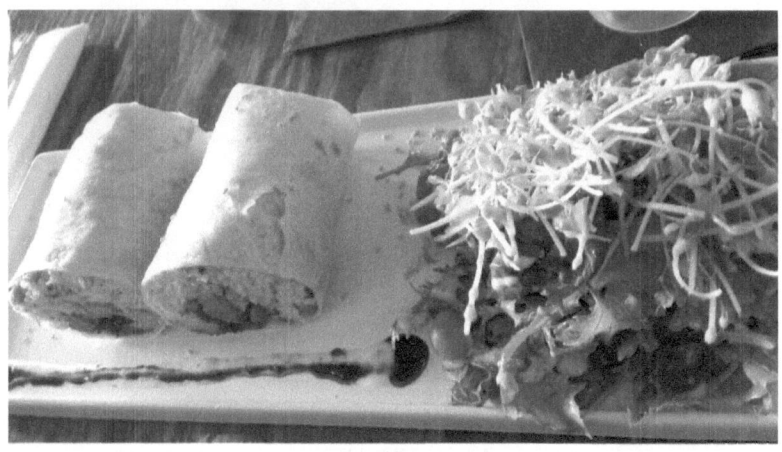

Here's a dish that you can take with you anywhere—it's easy
to make, too and will fulfill your barbecue cravings!

Yield: 4

Total Prep Time: 20 mins.

List of Ingredients:

- 2 cups baby spinach
- Four 8-inch whole wheat tortillas
- 1 cup canned black beans, drained and rinsed
- 1 cup frozen corn, thawed
- 8 oz chicken breast, sliced thinly
- 8 oz cooked steak, sliced thinly
- ½ cup low-fat cheese, shredded
- ¼ cup barbecue sauce

MMMMMMMMMMMMMMMMMMMMMMMMMMMMMMMMM

Methods:

1. Pre-heat the oven to 400 degrees then divide the corn, spinach, beans, steak and cheese among the tortillas.

2. Drizzle barbecue sauce over the tortillas and wrap the tortillas up.

3. Coat a baking dish lightly with cooking spray.

4. Place tortillas in the baking dish and heat for around 10 minutes.

5. Serve and enjoy!

(28) Stir-fried Chicken

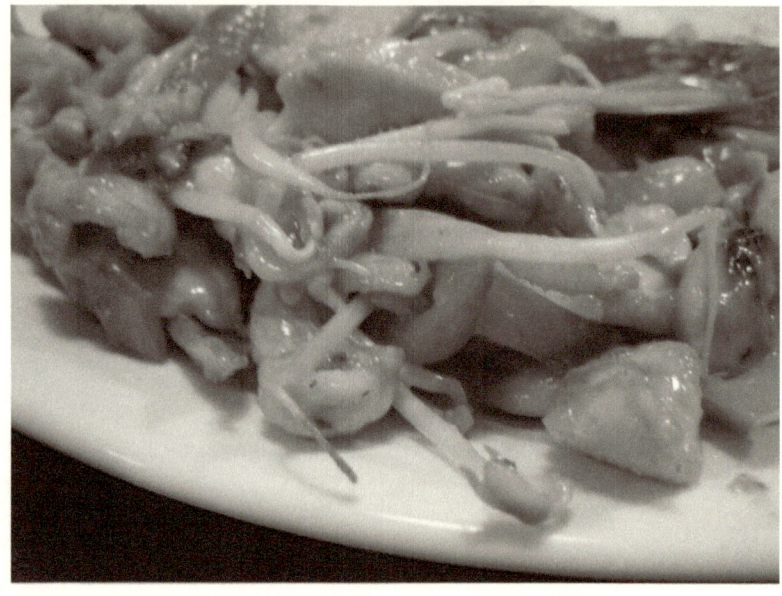

A terrific meal, that can go well with zucchini noodles and other vegetables.

Yield: 4

Total Prep Time: 50 mins.

List of Ingredients:

- 4 skinless and boneless chicken breasts
- 2 Tablespoons soy sauce
- 3 Tablespoons cornstarch
- ¼ teaspoons garlic powder
- ½ teaspoons ground ginger
- 1 cup celery, sliced
- 2 cups broccoli florets
- 1 small onion, cut into wedges
- 1 cup carrot, sliced thinly
- 3 Tablespoons cooking oil, divided
- 1 teaspoon chicken bouillon granule
- 1 cup water

MMMMMMMMMMMMMMMMMMMMMMMMMMMMMMM

Methods:

1. Cut chicken into strips then place the strips in a re-sealable bag. Add cornstarch and toss until well-coated.

2. Combine ginger, soy sauce and garlic powder in a bag then shake thoroughly and refrigerate for at least 30 minutes.

3. Heat 2 tablespoons of oil in a skillet then stir-fry the chicken until it is no longer pink or for at least 3 to 5 minutes. Remove from the skillet and make sure to keep warm.

4. Add water and the chicken bouillon granule then bring the chicken back to the pan. Cook until thick and bubbly.

5. Serve and enjoy!

(29) Ola Black Bean Salad

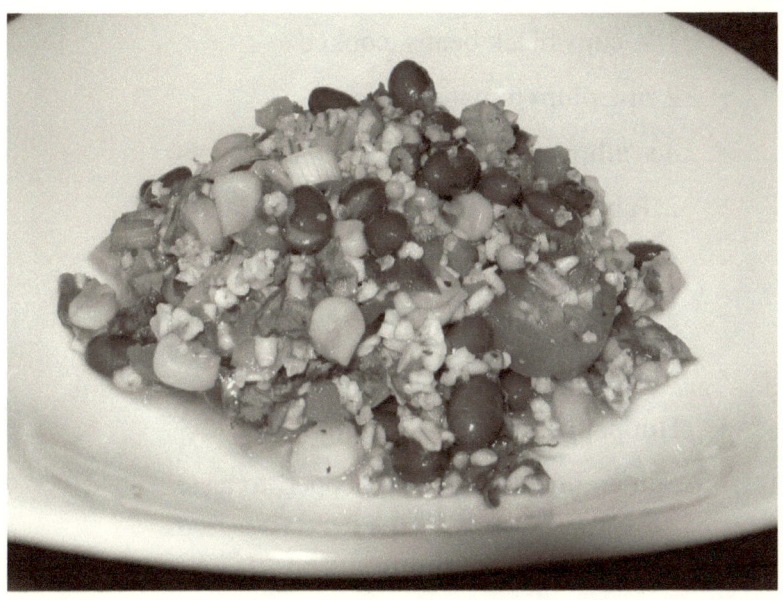

This salad is perfect for dinner because of its very low-calorie content and the fact that black beans are the healthiest and least arthritis/gout-inducing of all beans!

Yield: 4

Total Prep Time: 10 mins.

List of Ingredients:

- 1/3 cup canned corn
- 1 ½ cups black beans, cooked
- 2 ripe plum tomatoes, diced
- 3 scallions, sliced
- 2 Tablespoons freshly chopped cilantro
- 1 tablespoon fresh lime juice
- 2 Tablespoons olive oil
- Minced garlic
- Hot peppers
- Salt and freshly ground pepper, to taste

MMMMMMMMMMMMMMMMMMMMMMMMMMMMMMMMMM

Methods:

1. In a medium bowl, combine all of the ingredients and toss gently until well-combined. Refrigerate the salad until ready to serve.

2. Add parsley, peppers or any other herbs of your choice, if desired.

3. Serve and enjoy!

(30) Very Veggie Soup

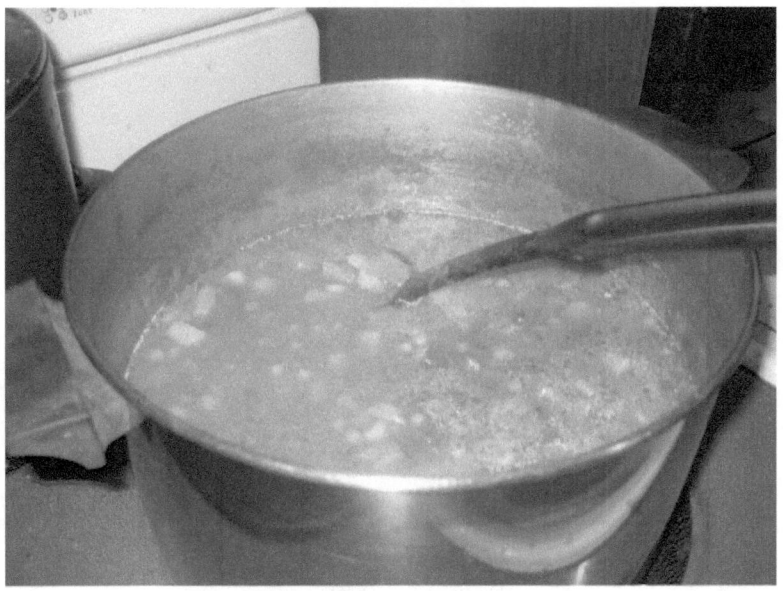

This soup has featured veggies galore! You can serve it up with crackers, croutons or a loaf of bread to round out the meal.

Yield: 4

Total Prep Time: 1 hr. 20 mins.

List of Ingredients:

- 1 medium carrot, peeled and chopped into small pieces
- 4 Tablespoons olive oil
- 1 tablespoon fresh ginger, grated
- 1 large potato, peeled and diced
- 2 cloves garlic, crushed
- 1 large onion, chopped
- 2 teaspoons salt
- 5 cups water
- 1 teaspoon cumin
- 1 teaspoon pepper
- 1 cup coriander leaves, chopped finely
- 4 medium tomatoes, chopped
- 1/8 teaspoons cayenne

MMMMMMMMMMMMMMMMMMMMMMMMMMMMMMMM

Methods:

1. In a saucepan, heat the oil then stir-fry the carrots together with garlic, onion and ginger for 5 minutes over medium heat.

2. Add tomatoes, coriander and potatoes then boil.

3. Simmer for around an hour in low heat, covered then add more water, if necessary.

4. Puree the mixture in a food processor then bring it back to the pan and make sure to heat before serving.

5. Enjoy!

About the Author

A native of Indianapolis, Indiana, Valeria Ray found her passion for cooking while she was studying English Literature at Oakland City University. She decided to try a cooking course with her friends and the experience changed her forever. She enrolled at the Art Institute of Indiana which offered extensive courses in the culinary Arts. Once Ray dipped her toe in the cooking world, she never looked back.

When Valeria graduated, she worked in French restaurants in the Indianapolis area until she became the head chef at one of the 5-star establishments in the area. Valeria's attention to taste and visual detail caught the eye of a local business person who expressed an interest in publishing her recipes. Valeria began her secondary career authoring cookbooks and e-books which she tackled with as much talent and gusto as her first career. Her passion for food leaps off the page of her books which have colourful anecdotes and stunning pictures of dishes she has prepared herself.

Valeria Ray lives in Indianapolis with her husband of 15 years, Tom, her daughter, Isobel and their loveable Golden Retriever, Goldy. Valeria enjoys cooking special dishes in her large, comfortable kitchen where the family gets involved in preparing meals. This successful, dynamic chef is an inspiration to culinary students and novice cooks everywhere.

•••••••••• ● ● ● ● ● ● ● •••••••

Author's Afterthoughts

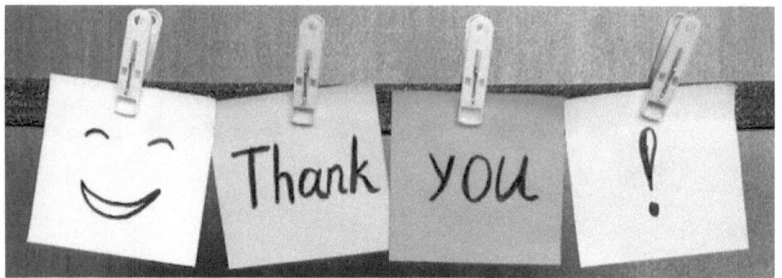

Thank you for Purchasing my book and taking the time to read it from front to back. I am always grateful when a reader chooses my work and I hope you enjoyed it!

With the vast selection available online, I am touched that you chose to be purchasing my work and take valuable time out of your life to read it. My hope is that you feel you made the right decision.

I very much would like to know what you thought of the book. Please take the time to write an honest and informative review on Amazon.com. Your experience and opinions will be of great benefit to me and those readers looking to make an informed choice.

With much thanks,

Valeria Ray

www.ingramcontent.com/pod-product-compliance
Lightning Source LLC
Chambersburg PA
CBHW020339290526
45785CB00005B/2085